INFUSIONS:

10 Simple Infused Water Recipes To Make Your Water Taste Great and Live Healthier (Fruit Infused Water Recipes, Water Infusion Recipes)

By: Kendall Woods

result of the use of information contained within this document, including, but not limited to, —errors, omissions, or inaccuracies.

Contents

Introduction

Let me start off by expressing how happy it makes to me to see that you have chosen to download and read my book!

Water is perhaps the most fundamental and basic building block upon which every single living organism exists. Where there is water, there is life.

Even though the gravity and importance of water in our day to day life is unparalleled. There are a whole lot of individuals who perceive water as being a very bland and ordinary drink. In doing so, generally they tend to avoid regular water and go for caffeinated beverages such as coffee or tea or even carbonated beverages to keep the body hydrated.

While these "processed" liquids do in fact help to keep the body hydrated, they do that while exposing the body to an unfathomable amount of sugar which greatly amps up to affect the normal bodily functions and produce adverse conditions. Not to mention increased weight that leads to obesity!

Water Infused recipes are like a blessing for those individual. As with these, they will be able to both fulfill their desire for a delicious mouthwatering (literally) flavor while supplying the body with a healthy punch of nutrients and vitamins!

Consumption of Infused Water has risen to a large scope recently and now has encouraged thousands of people all around the world to clean up their personal bottles and containers to prepare themselves for a unique journey.

Infused water recipes are popping up every now and then in various websites, social media adverts.

The aim of this book is to help you understand the core concepts of Water Infused drinks and give you a kick start on this journey!

The book not only comes with a detailed and elaborate discussion of a Water Infused Diet, but also is packed with 10 unique and delicious recipes that are ready to improve your health in no time and open up a whole new world of liquid possibilities for you!

Chapter 1
Getting to Know About Infused Water

All of a sudden the hype surrounding the topic of Water Infusion has expanded to a massive size. Not only because of all of the health properties it has, but also because of how effective it is when it comes to trimming down your fat and help you attain that beautiful body which you have been dreaming of!

But even today, there are thousands and thousands of people who are unaware of the plethora of positive effects that can be acquire through the consumption of Infused Water. Even more, there are people who are completely unaware of the existence of this form of diet!

The first chapter of this book is going to be dedicated for those individuals who are looking at this topic for the first time ever!

What exactly is "Infused Water"?

The fun thing here is that by now you probably have already tried infused water without even being aware of it!

You have probably heard of Detox water right? The liquid mixtures that are used to get rid of the harmful toxins from our body? Well, that is basically Infused Water!

For a more strict definition, any "body" of water that has been properly processed to have the flavors of fruits or vegetables induced in its liquid is referred to as "Infused Water"

These can range from the aforementioned detox water, to water that is naturally flavored by a fruit.

These drinks are not only suitable for your personal use, but can also be used at any parties or ceremonies to light up the mood and re-energize the lost vigor of your guests!

You know what the best part is? You will be getting the flavors of your favorite soda without any of the calories!

The positive effects of Infused Water

Now that you know a bit about Infused water, next you are definitely curious to know what the benefits of consuming Infused Water are. Well, honestly listing the benefits that can be obtained from an Infused Water diet will just keep on going and going until my electronic ink runs out! However, for your convenience, I am going to be listing out some of the more prominent ones!

Keeping your body hydrated throughout the day is undoubtedly the prime benefit of consuming infused water. With our busy lifestyle, it has become really hard for us to maintain the required 64 ounce of water consumption and stay healthy. But then again, we are always getting time for soft drinks right?

Flavor is a very important factor here. The reason why we are so much inclined towards drinking carbonated beverages is because they are flavored as such. On the other hand, pure water is just tasteless!

So, the very first benefit which you may have already thought of, is the fact that having a glass of water filled with the flavors of a number of fruits and vegetables will naturally encourage you to drink more water throughout the day!

But there's more! Aside from being hydrated, you will also be able to enjoy the benefits of the different ingredients that you use to prepare you water.

- With infused water, you are getting a very healthy dose of required Anti-Oxidants, Vitamins and Minerals to satisfy the needs of your body.

- Since you are always experimenting different kinds of ingredients, the ability of an infused drink to cast off diseases might vary from drink to drink. But, In general they range from lowering the body's proneness towards diabetes, cold, heart disease, and flu. Since all of the ingredients used in infused water are natural compounds, they also help you to a great extent to protect the body from Cancer!

- With the rich levels of antioxidants in this infused waters, you will be able to substantially slow down the aging effect and fend off any radical damage. Thanks to the increased production of collagen, infused drinks helps to make the skin much more smooth!

- This one is more related towards weight loss. The active compounds present in various fruits helps to significantly increase the body's metabolism speed which helps it to burn more calories in a day

- If you are looking for a burst of energy, then these drinks are the way to go! Since these drinks are packed with a large amount of vitamins, they are able to keep you energized all throughout the day, non-stop! Making these ideal for individuals who explore a more active lifestyle such as fitness buffs or athletes.

- The junk food all around us may cause our body to suffer from bloated tummy or gas or any other digestion issues. If you are also a sufferer, then an Infused Water is here to help you! Waters that are infused with Citrus have been shown to greatly enhance the digestive strength and aid to settle down your stomach problems. Alternatively, ginger, orange, apple, or papaya might help you to tackle your digestive problems while sending a cooling sensation down your stomach.

- Since these drinks are packed with antioxidants it helps to fully cleanse out the toxins of your body. Not only will this keep you hydrated, but will also strengthen your immune system!

- Are you a sweet tooth but can't go for delicious savories because of calories? Just go ahead and stir up a nice infused drink to satisfy that sweet thirst of yours while making sure that you are exposed to only a few calories at max!

Chapter 2
Recipes Galore

Rosemary and Strawberry Detox Water

(For 2 liter serving)

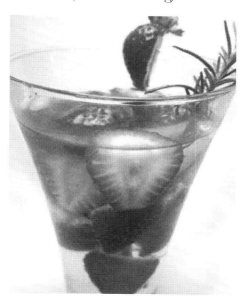

If you are looking for a drink to fully detoxify your body, then you can't go wrong with this subtle mixture of Rosemary and Strawberry. This drink will not only enhance your overall health, but will also increase your cranial functions.

If you are not aware of it, then you should know that amongst the healthiest herbs out there, Rosemary stands amongst the top!

Rosemary has been used for ages to treat muscular pain, strengthen the immune system, improve cognitive functions as well as improve the conditions of the circulatory system.

Rosemary is packed with anti-inflammatory chemicals which also helps the body defend itself from severe asthma attacks.

Not only that! Rosemary also aids largely in mitigating various digestion problems involving heartburn and gas. Amongst the various diseases and symptoms, Rosemary has been proven to be highly effective in dealing with cough, gout, headache, memory issues and high blood pressure.

Rosemary is not the only hero of the show though! Strawberries are also fantastic carriers of a bunch of anti-oxidants like Vitamin C and helps to relief the body from symptoms of cancer, stroke and heart diseases.

Together with these two ingredients, this drink is a complete powerhouse that is both delicious and invigorating.

Ingredients:

- 2-3 sprigs of fresh rosemary
- 15 pieces of quartered strawberry
- 2 full cups of ice
- Water as required

Preparation:

1. The first step here is to take a large sized pitcher and toss in the strawberries and rosemary.

2. Fill up the container with the ice and pour in water.

3. Store the pitcher inside your fridge and let it cool there for about an hour.

4. Once the drink has reached its desired temperature, take it out and pour about ¾ or the pitcher in another glass and it is ready to serve.

5. Fill up the original pitcher again and store it in the fridge.

6. Keep repeating for as long as you want. Strawberry and Rosemary Detox water can be stored in the fridge for a maximum of 24 hours.

Tropical Pineapple and Orange Infused Water

(For 2 liter serving)

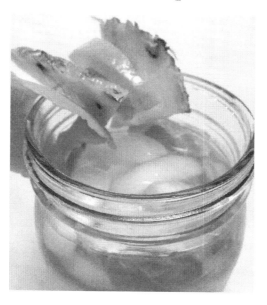

Missing that wonderful sea beach experience of last year? Want to go there and indulge yourself under the sun once again but just don't have enough time? Well, look no further and conjure yourself up a batch of this mighty fine Tropical Pineapple and Orange Infused Water cocktail.

Just a few sips from this drink will make you feel like you are finally enjoying yourself a day at the beach!

This drink is a fine amalgam of a vivid tropical flavor which is balanced out by the sweetness of this drink.

Pineapples and Oranges, the two core ingredients of this recipe are both superb holders of Vitamin C!

Amongst the various health benefits of this drink, some include:

- Help in digestion
- Strengthening of Immune System.
- Enhance body regeneration
- Works as a powerful anti-inflammatory agent.

Ingredients:

- 1 thinly sliced orange
- ½ a cup of thinly slice pineapple
- 2 full cups of ice
- Water as needed

Preparation:

1. Here you are going to start this recipe by taking a large sized pitcher and toss in the pineapple and orange slices.
2. Fill up the container with the ice and pour in water.
3. Store the pitcher inside your fridge and let it cool for about an hour.

4. Once the drink has reached its desired temperature, take it out and pour about ¾ of the pitcher in another glass and drink it up.

5. Fill up the original pitcher again and store it in the fridge.

6. Keep repeating it for as long as you want. Tropical Pineapple and orange infused pitcher can be stored in the fridge for a maximum of 24 hours.

Lemon Water with Blueberries and Mint

(For 2 liter serving)

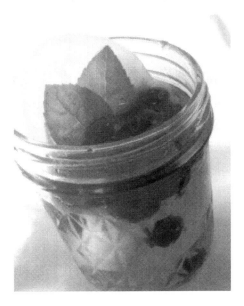

This is a recipe that is particularly jam packed with a delightful collection of multiple antioxidants and vitamins. Not to mention, this is a highly effective vigor for individuals who are interested in losing weight as well!

Due to the high potency of Vitamin C in this drink, this drink helps to regulate the hormones which influence the storage of fat that further helps to lose fat more easily.

Blueberries are known as an Anti-Inflammatory Super Food and are also known to vastly improve heart conditions and tackle cancerous cells.

The lemon in this recipe is responsible for maintaining a good weight and improve your whole digestive system.

On the other hand, the inclusion of Mint is what helps to primarily lose your weight by raising your overall bodily energy and help you burn up calories with ease.

Ingredients:

- 1 piece of thinly sliced lemon
- 1 cup of blueberries
- 10 pieces of mint leaves
- 2 full cups of ice
- Water as needed

Preparation:

1. Take a large sized pitcher and toss in the blueberries and lemon.
2. On top of the lemon and blueberries, squeeze and twist your mints making sure that they are not torn apart.
3. The main objective here is to gently release the oil.
4. Once enough oil is out, toss in the mint leaves to the fruits as well.
5. Fill up the container with the ice and pour in water.
6. Store the pitcher inside your fridge and let it cool there for about an hour.
7. Once the drink has reached its desired temperature, take it out and pour about ¾ or the pitcher in another glass and drink it up.
8. Fill up the original pitcher again and store it in the fridge.
9. Keep repeating it for as long as you want. Lemon Water and Blueberry can be stored in the fridge for a maximum of 24 hours.

Ginger and Mango Infused Water

(For 2 liter serving)

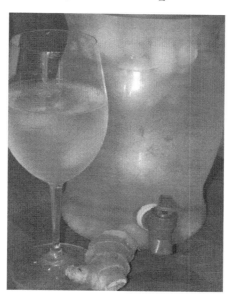

This fine recipe takes the health benefits of ginger and combines it with the sweetness of Mango to mask down the sometimes tingling flavor of Ginger.

The ginger in particular in this recipe helps to a great extent as a natural painkiller for migraines.

If you have the tendency of suffering from motion sickness or heartburn, it will also help you with this.

Aside from making this drink a delight, the Mango helps to boost up the bodily metabolism and help your body digest food better.

Ingredients:

- A peeled and sliced up ginger root of 1 inch in size
- 1 cup of either fresh or frozen mango

Preparation:

1. Start off this recipe by processing the ginger. Take a vegetable peeler and peel out the part which you are going to use.

2. After that, take a knife and slice up just about 3-4 pieces of coin sized portions.

3. Take a pitcher and toss in the mango and processed Ginger slices.

4. Fill up the container with about 3 cups of ice and then pour in the water.

5. Make sure that the ginger is firmly pressed down by the ice.

6. Place the drink inside your fridge for about 2-3 hours

7. Take it out and toss in some frozen mango chunks and serve.

8. The drink can be stored in the fridge for about 24 hours

Cooling Peach and Mint Water

(For 2 liter serving)

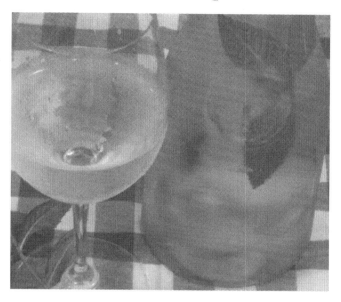

Summer is just around the corner and the time of facing the burning heat of the sun is soon approaching!

You are going to need something to tackle this heat so that you don't dehydrate!

The aim of this drink is precisely that!

The mint in this drink alongside the water acts as a natural air conditioner to nicely cool your whole body while helping you to lose a couple of pounds as well, thanks to the peaches.

This is a very reinvigorating combination to refresh you whenever you like.

And if you think that the drink is not sweet enough, then just go ahead and toss in a couple of extra peach slices and just a dash of vanilla for a more intense flavor

Ingredients:

- 1 long Sprig Mint
- 10 pieces of Frozen Peach Slices
- Water as required
- Ice as required

Preparation:

1. The first step here is to take a moderately sized pitcher and toss in the peaches

2. Then toss in the mint leaves

3. Toss in all of the ice and top everything off and pour in the water

4. Place the pitcher in your fridge for at least 4 hours or keep it stored overnight.

5. Take a nice wine glass and serve the drink

6. If you prefer, garnish it with some frozen peach slices

7. Once all of the water runs out, you can fill up the pitcher again and keep repeating it for 8 times.

Fall Fruit Infused Water with Pears, Cranberries and Clementine

(For 2 liter serving)

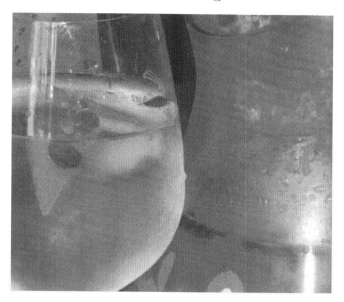

When the air starts to get cooler and the trees start to change their color, it's the certain indication that fall is approaching soon.

Which means the start of the next season of the TV series you watch and the football season is coming soon!

This drink is hand prepared for such a unique occasion. The multiple layers of flavors makes this healthy, delicious and also supremely refreshing!

Upon sipping this drink, you will first be greeted by a tingling sensation from the allspice berries that will be soon be overtaken by the tender sweetness of the clementine and pears.

Ingredients:

- 1 piece of thinly sliced pear

- 1 piece of Clementine Orange cut into 8 small pieces

- 1 tablespoon of Dried Cranberries

- 1 teaspoon of All Spice Berries

Preparation:

1. Take a large sized pitcher and toss in the ingredients.

2. Cover it with ice and pour in just enough water to cover it half way

3. Once done, keep the water inside the fridge and let it freeze for at 3 hours before serving

4. If the water runs out, then you can refill it once again. And it can be repeated for 3-5 times before needing to replace the contents again

Apple Cinnamon Water

(For 2 liter serving)

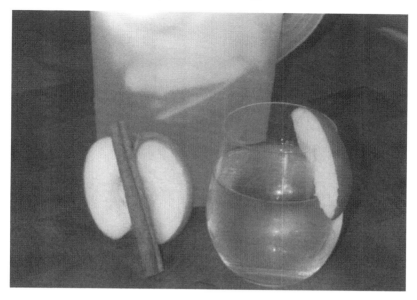

We all know the health benefits of apple! It is as they say.

"An apple a day, keeps the doctor away!"

So why not make an infused recipe out of it?

Not only will you be getting all of the health benefits of apple here, but thanks to the combination of apple with Cinnamon, you will have a much sturdier and faster metabolic rate in your body!

Just a piece of advice, for this recipe you might want to look into Honey crisp or Fuji apples as they will give you the most delicious drink. And, if you are in the mood for a little more flavor, then add in the some more slices of apple.

Ingredients:

- 1 thinly sliced piece of Apple of your choosing
- 1 Cinnamon Stick

Preparation:

1. Take a large sized pitcher and toss in the apple slices to the bottom of the pitcher

2. Toss in the cinnamon stick

3. Cover it with ice and pour in just enough water to cover it half way

4. Once done, keep the water inside the fridge and let it cool for at least 1 hour before serving

5. If the water runs out, then you can refill it once again. And it can be repeated for 3-4 times before needing to replace the contents again.

Detox Lime Cucumber Mint Water

(For 2 liter serving)

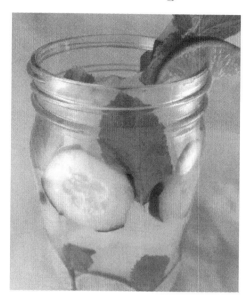

Getting rid of all the pollutants from your body is extremely important once in awhile to make sure that the body is functioning properly in the long run!

This Detoxifying drink won't only help you to detox your body of all the wastage, but also give you a nice burst of freshness

The cucumber alongside the mint here acts as a strong anti-inflammatory duo which helps you to reduce a bloated tummy while being injected with a plethora of Vitamin C from the lime.

Ingredients:

- 1 thinly sliced lime
- 1 piece of 5 inch cucumber sliced into ring shapes
- 5 pieces of mint leaves
- 2 full cups of ice
- Water as required

Preparation:

1. The first step here is to take a moderately sized pitcher and toss in the lime and cucumber

2. Over the lime and cucumber, twist and squeeze the lime making sure that you don't tear it apart. Just the oil needs to be gently released

3. Add in the mint to the pitcher then

4. Toss in all of the ice and top everything off and pour in the water

5. Place the pitcher in your fridge for at least 4 hours or keep it stored overnight.

6. Take a nice wine glass and serve the drink

7. If you prefer, then garnish it with some frozen peach slices

8. Once all of the water runs out, you can fill up the pitcher again and keep repeating it for 3-5 times.

Lavender Lemonade

(For 2 liter serving)

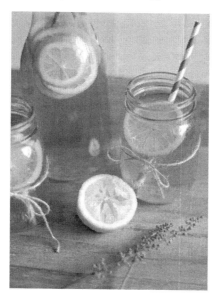

We all love lemonades right? But going for the traditional lemonade is just way too overrated and mainstream these days!

And exactly for that reason, I have brought you a fine Lemonade recipe that is sure to turn you into the talk of the day around your neighborhood.

Be prepared that this recipe will require you to go just a little bit beyond the normal twisting and squeezing! But rest assured, you won't be disappointed with the results.

Ingredients:

Ingredients for Lavender Mix

- 2 cups of water
- ½ a cup of sugar
- ¼ cup of honey
- 3 tablespoon of dried lavender

Ingredients for the Lemonade

- 2 cups of freshly squeezed lemon juice
- 4 cups of water
- 1 sliced lemon

Preparation:

1. The first step here is to prepare your syrup. You can do that by taking a saucepan over medium heat and pour in about 2 cups of water and the sugar

2. Bring the mixture to boil and keep whisking it until the sugar has been fully dissolved

3. Turn off the heat and stir in the honey and pieces of dried lavender

4. Keep in covered about 15 minutes, letting the mixture to finely steep.

5. Finely strain the lavender under pressure to make sure that all of the juices are released

6. Take a large sized pitcher and combine the previously prepared lavender mixture with water and lemon juice

7. Add a few drops of coloring of your choice

8. Store it in the fridge for at least 2 hours and serve it fully chilled!

Strawberry Jalapeno

(For 32 ounce Ball Jar)

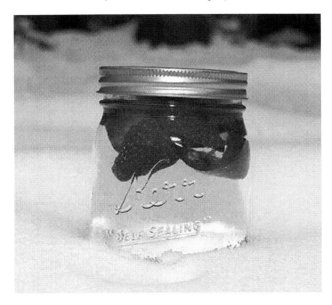

Up until this point, all of the recipes have been mostly sweet filled infusions.

I would like to end this book on a spicy note with this Jalapeno infused drink!

So, if you are looking for a drink that will turn you into a fire breathing dragon, this is the one to go for!

The Jalapeno in this recipe will help you to bring on the heat while the strawberries will provide a hint of sweetness.

Keep in mind that ½ of a Jalapeno pepper will produce a significantly spicy drink! However, if you want to lower down the flame, then go for about ¼ of a pepper.

Ingredients:

- 3 pieces of Organic Strawberries
- ½ of a jalapeno pepper
- Ice as required
- Water as required

Preparation:

1. The first step here is to prepare your strawberries by cutting off the top area
2. Slice them into two halves
3. Take a plastic wrap and use it to wrap over your finger and de-seed the Jalapeno
4. Take a large sized pitcher and toss in the ingredients
5. Fill it up with cold water and let it sit inside the fridge for about 3-4 hours
6. Enjoy the spicy chill!

Conclusion

Once again I would like to thank you for purchasing the book and taking the time for going through the book as well.

I do hope that this book has been helpful and you found the information contained within useful!

Here at The Purest Drop, we believe that everyone deserves to have access to clean drinking water. We partner up with charities to provide safe, clean drinkable water in developing countries. We sell refrigerator water filters to you, providing you with the clean water you need. With a portion of the proceeds, we donate to help provide clean drinking water to those who need it most.

Join us in making a difference, one drop at a time…

Get $5 any of our products on Amazon using the coupon code: **FIVETPDR**

http://amzn.to/2h58QgY

To learn more about us visit our website:

ThePurestDrop.com

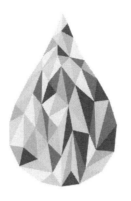

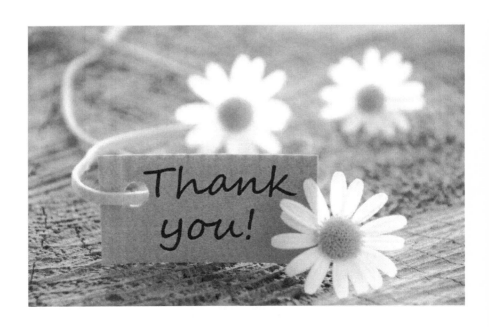

77498002R00024

Made in the USA
Middletown, DE
21 June 2018